BULIMIA NERVO:
BOC

A Cookbook for Those Struggling with Bulimia Nervosa: Recipes and Important Advice

REX LEWIS

Table of Contents

Introduction

The hallmark of bulimia nervosa is recurring episodes of binge eating, which are followed by compensatory actions meant to avoid weight gain. Bulimia sufferers frequently partake in self-inflicted vomiting, abuse laxatives or diuretics, fasting, or over exercise.

Key Characteristics Of Bulimia Nervosa Consist Of:

1. Binge Eating: People who suffer from bulimia have periods of extreme food intake that usually last only a short while. During these episodes, they often feel like they have no control over their eating.

2. Compensatory actions: People with bulimia participate in compensatory actions to offset the possible weight gain from binge eating. Self-induced vomiting, overexertion, starvation, or improper use of drugs such as diuretics or laxatives are a few examples of this.

3. Body Image Issues: Bulimia sufferers frequently have a distorted perception of their bodies and overemphasize their shapes and weight when judging their own value. Even if they are underweight, they could think of themselves as overweight.

4. Shame and Secrecy: Bulimia is frequently linked to feelings of shame and secrecy. People will often go to considerable measures in order to conceal their eating habits and the results of their compensatory acts.

5. Medical And Psychological Consequences: Electrolyte imbalances, gastrointestinal disorders, dental problems, anxiety, depression, and social isolation are just a few of the medical and psychological problems that bulimia can cause.

6. The onset and progression of bulimia nervosa are usually associated with adolescence or early adulthood. If treatment is not received, the disease may worsen with time, although recovery is achievable with the right measures.

7. Diagnostic Standards: In accordance with the Diagnostic and Statistical Manual of Mental Disorders (DSM-5), an individual cannot be diagnosed with bulimia nervosa unless certain diagnostic standards are satisfied.

A multidisciplinary strategy is frequently used in the treatment of bulimia nervosa, encompassing dietary counseling, psychotherapy (such as cognitive-behavioral therapy), and, in certain situations, medication. Having the support of friends and family is essential to the healing process.

It should be emphasized that receiving expert assistance is necessary for both diagnosis and therapy. It is advised that you get in touch with a medical practitioner or mental health provider if you believe that you or someone you know is experiencing bulimia or any other eating disorder.

CHAPTER ONE
Defined Terms and Diagnostic Standards

Mental health practitioners frequently utilize the Diagnostic and Statistical Manual of Mental illnesses, Fifth Edition (DSM-5) to diagnose psychiatric illnesses, and it contains the diagnostic criteria for bulimia nervosa. The DSM-5 states that in order to be diagnosed with bulimia nervosa, a person must fulfill the following requirements:

• **Repeated Bouts of Binge Eating:** The individual has repeated episodes of binge eating, which are defined by eating a quantity of food that is noticeably more than what most people would eat in a comparable amount of time under comparable conditions. These episodes are also accompanied with a feeling of being out of control.

• **Frequent Improper Compensatory Behaviors:** The person frequently self-induces vomiting, abuses laxatives, diuretics, or other drugs, fasts, or participates in excessive activity in an attempt to prevent weight gain.

• For three months, binge eating and inappropriate compensatory behaviors must occur at least once a week on average. During that time, the binge eating and compensatory behaviors must occur at least once a week.

• Body type and weight unnecessarily impact self-evaluation: A person's body type and weight unduly influence their self-evaluation. The desire to maintain a particular weight or body type is persistent, and these things have a big effect on self-esteem.

• The disruption is not limited to periods of anorexia nervosa: The behaviors are not limited to anorexia nervosa episodes, in which the person severely restricts their food intake, resulting in abnormally low body weight.

It is crucial to remember that a mental health expert, such as a psychiatrist or psychologist, should perform a thorough examination before making a diagnosis. This assessment should take into account the patient's medical history, symptoms, and other pertinent information. A person with bulimia nervosa can greatly improve their prognosis with early intervention and adequate therapy.

Reasons and Danger Elements

A number of factors, including genetic, biochemical, psychological, and environmental ones, can contribute to the development of bulimia nervosa. Because of the intricate interactions between these components, pinpointing the precise cause might be difficult. The following are some known triggers and risk factors for the emergence of bulimia nervosa:

1. Genetic Factors: Research indicates that eating disorders, such as bulimia nervosa, may have a hereditary basis. A higher risk may apply to those with a family history of eating disorders or other mental health issues.

2. Biological Factors: The regulation of mood and hunger has been linked to specific neurotransmitters, such as serotonin, which are chemical messengers in the brain. Bulimia nervosa may arise as a result of imbalances in these neurotransmitters.

3. Psychological Factors: Perfectionism, impulsivity, low self-esteem, and trouble managing emotions are personality qualities that might lead to the development of bulimia nervosa. Another prevalent psychological cause is a skewed body image and body dissatisfaction.

4. Environmental Factors: Eating disorders can arise as a result of societal and cultural pressures around beauty standards, body image, and weight loss. Idealized body types that are shown in the media can have an impact on people, particularly in adolescence and early adulthood.

5. Traumatic Experiences: Neglect, abuse, or other traumatic events during childhood may increase the likelihood that bulimia nervosa would develop. These encounters may exacerbate issues with controlling one's emotions.

6. Diets and Weight-Related Behaviors: Excessive exercise, weight control methods, or severe diets can all be risk factors for developing bulimia nervosa. These actions could be brought on by personal conceptions of the ideal body type or by social influences.

7. Stress and Life Transitions: In susceptible individuals, bulimia nervosa may begin as a result of stressful life events, transitions, or significant life changes. Under stress, coping strategies involving food and body image may be impacted.

8.Cultural and Peer Influences: Bulimia nervosa may arise as a result of exposure to peers who engage in disordered eating practices or as a result of society's emphasis on thinness.

It is noteworthy that the relationship between these variables is intricate, and not every person who possesses risk factors will experience the onset of bulimia nervosa. Furthermore, the risk might be reduced by the existence of protective factors including robust social support and effective coping mechanisms. Effective t reatment and recovery depend heavily on early discovery and intervention. It's advised to get professional assistance if you or someone you know is dealing with bulimia or any other eating issue.

Symptoms and Indications

A person with bulimia nervosa may exhibit a variety of indications and symptoms in their behavior, emotions, and physical well-being. It's crucial to remember that bulimia sufferers may try to conceal their symptoms, making the illness difficult to identify. The following are typical indications and manifestations of bulimia nervosa:

1. Episodes of Binge Eating:

• Overindulging in food for a brief period of time, frequently experiencing moments of controllessness.

• During binges, eating a lot at once.

• Consuming food even when not truly hungry.

• Eating by themselves because they feel self-conscious about how much food they are consuming.

2. Reimbursing Actions:

• Post-meal self-inflicted vomiting.

- Abusing laxatives, diuretics, or other drugs in an attempt to lose weight.

- Strict dieting or fasting.

- Excessive physical activity, even while hurt or in bad weather.

3. Disorder of the Body Image:

- Strong unhappiness with the shape or size of one's physique.

- A skewed perception of one's body, perceiving oneself as overweight even when underweight.

4. Symptoms in the body:

• Swollen or painful glands, particularly in the jaw region (caused by recurrent vomiting).

• Russell's sign, which is a callus or scar on the hands or knuckles from self-induced vomiting.

• Dental issues include cavities, sensitivity, or erosion of the enamel.

• Digestive problems, including constipation, bloating, or irregular bowel motions.

5. Signs of the mind and emotions:

• Sadness or anxiety.

• An obsession with weight, diets, and eating.

• Variations in mood.

• Low self-worth and guilty or ashamed sentiments, especially following binge eating episodes.

6. Behavioral and Social Shifts:

• Refusing to participate in social gatherings or culinary-related events.

• An overemphasis on mealtime rituals and food preparation.

· Secrecy regarding behavior or eating habits.

7. Modifications to the Body:

• Variations in weight, frequently falling into the normal or marginally above-average range.

• Weakness and exhaustion.

• Lightheadedness or dizziness.

8. Irregularities in menstruation:

• For females, absentee menstruation (amenorrhea) or irregular menstrual cycles.

It's important to understand that symptoms can vary in severity and that not everyone with bulimia nervosa will show all of these indicators. It is crucial to get professional assistance from a healthcare provider, therapist, or eating disorder specialist if you believe that you or someone you know is experiencing bulimia nervosa. This will ensure an accurate diagnosis and the right course of therapy. The likelihood of recovery can be considerably increased with early intervention.

CHAPTER TWO
The Effects of Bulimia on Health

Bulimia nervosa can have serious health effects on the body that impact several organ systems. Physical and psychological issues may arise from the recurrent cycles of binge eating and compensatory behaviors. It's crucial to remember that each person will experience health problems to varying degrees, some of which could be fatal. The following are a few negative health effects of bulimia nervosa:

1. Digestive Disorders:

• Recurrent vomiting can cause the esophagus to become inflamed and irritated, which can lead to esophageal tears or ruptures.

Heartburn and gastric reflux are frequently caused by the stomach acids that are regurgitated during vomiting.

- There could be bleeding in the stomach.

2. Electrolyte Disproportions:

- Abnormalities in the amounts of potassium, sodium, chloride, and other vital electrolytes might result from frequent vomiting and laxative use, which can upset the electrolyte balance.

• Serious side effects from electrolyte imbalances include cardiac arrhythmias, convulsions, and, in the worst situations, heart failure.

3. Dental Problems:

• Stomach acid exposure while vomiting can erode tooth enamel, resulting in gum disease, cavities, and sensitivity.

• Regular vomiting may cause the telltale "Russell's sign," as well as calluses or scars on the hands or knuckles from coming into contact with teeth during vomiting induction.

4. Complications Related To The Heart:

• Dehydration and electrolyte imbalances can put a strain on the cardiovascular system, raising the risk of cardiac arrest and perhaps causing palpitations and abnormal heart rhythms.

5. The reproductive and endocrine systems:

• Menstrual abnormalities, such as amenorrhea (lack of menstruation), can occur in bulimic women.

• Bone density and reproductive health may be impacted by hormonal abnormalities.

6. Inadequate Dietary Resources:

• Deficits in vital vitamins and minerals might result from vomiting, laxative use, or restricted meals, which can impair immune system and general health.

7. Kidney and Renal Complications:

• renal injury or failure can result from electrolyte imbalances and dehydration's impact on renal function.

8. Osteoskeletal Problems:

• Loss of bone density (osteoporosis), tiredness, and

muscle weakness can be caused by overexertion and poor nutrition.

9. Psychiatric Repercussions:

• Anxiety, sadness, and other mental health problems can be exacerbated by bulimia's psychological effects and chronic physical stress.

10. Heightened Likelihood Of Co-Occurring Disorders

• People who struggle with bulimia are more likely to experience additional mental health issues such substance abuse, anxiety disorders, and depression.

It's critical to get professional assistance for bulimia nervosa diagnosis and treatment. A multidisciplinary approach is usually used in treatment, involving nutritional, psychological, and medicinal therapies. Mitigating the health effects and fostering recuperation necessitate early intervention. Seek help from a medical practitioner or eating disorder specialist if you or someone you know is exhibiting signs of bulimia nervosa.

Asking For Assistance

Getting treatment is essential for recovery if you or someone you know is exhibiting signs of an eating disorder, such as bulimia nervosa. The following actions are things to think about:

1. Speak with a Medical Professional:

• Speak with a medical expert first, such as a registered dietician, psychiatrist, or primary care physician. To ascertain the extent of the eating disorder and any related health issues, they can do an evaluation.

2. Psychological Assessment:

• To evaluate the emotional and mental components of bulimia nervosa, a psychological examination can be performed by a mental health expert, such as a psychologist, psychiatrist, or clinical social worker.

3. Team for Treatment:

• Put together a treatment team that might include medical specialists, therapists, and nutritionists who specialize in eating disorders. Complete support is offered through collaborative care.

4. Counseling and Therapy:

• Research has demonstrated that bulimia nervosa can be effectively treated with cognitive-behavioral therapy (CBT). Additional treatment modalities, such interpersonal therapy or dialectical behavior therapy (DBT), might also be helpful.

5. Dietary Advice:

• Consult with a nutritionist or licensed dietitian with expertise in eating problems. They can offer direction on forming wholesome eating habits and taking care of nutritional deficits.

6. Drugs:

• Medication may occasionally be recommended to treat particular symptoms or co-occurring illnesses like anxiety or depression.

7. Support Teams:

• Participating in an online or in-person support group helps foster understanding and a sense of community. Organizations that specialize in eating disorders or mental health professionals might lead support groups.

8. Include Friends and Family:

• Inform and include loved ones in the process of becoming well. It can help to have a social network that is encouraging.

9. In-patient Care or Comprehensive Therapy Plans:

• Admission to the hospital or enrollment in rigorous outpatient or inpatient treatment programs may be required in extreme circumstances or when there are substantial health risks.

10. Continue Getting Regular Checkups at the Med:

• To monitor physical health and handle any medical issues related to bulimia nervosa, routine medical check-ups are essential.

Recall that asking for assistance is a sign of strength and that, with the right care and support, recovery is achievable. If you don't know where to begin, think about getting in touch with hotlines, eating disorder helplines, or mental health groups. For information and support, call the National Eating Disorders Association (NEDA) Helpline (1-800-931-2237) in the US. Similar tools might be accessible through regional mental health organizations in other nations.

Options for Treatment

Bulimia nervosa is usually treated with a multidisciplinary approach that takes into account the disorder's dietary, psychological, and physical components. The exact course of treatment may change depending on the needs of each patient, the intensity of their symptoms, and the existence of any co-occurring disorders. The following are typical elements of bulimia nervosa treatment:

1. Psychoanalysis:

- Cognitive-Behavioral Therapy (CBT): The most extensively studied and empirically supported kind of psychotherapy for bulimia nervosa is CBT. It focuses on recognizing and altering eating- and body-image-related cognitive patterns and behaviors.

- Dialectical Behavior Therapy (DBT): Addressing emotional regulation, interpersonal effectiveness, and distress tolerance, DBT may be helpful for people who suffer from bulimia.

• Interpersonal psychotherapy (IPT): IPT examines how interpersonal connections and communication abilities may either influence or be impacted by an eating disorder. Its main goal is to improve these areas.

2. Dietary Advice:

• Consult with a nutritionist or licensed dietitian who specializes in eating disorders. In addition to addressing nutritional shortages and promoting good eating habits, they can assist in establishing regular and balanced eating patterns.

3. Drugs:

- Selective Serotonin Reuptake Inhibitors (SSRIs): To help control mood and lessen binge-purge tendencies, doctors may prescribe antidepressant drugs, especially SSRIs like fluoxetine (Prozac).

- Individual requirements and factors should be taken into account when making medication decisions, which should be discussed with a psychiatrist or other mental health expert.

4. Medical Surveillance:

- To monitor physical health, evaluate the effects of bulimia on the body, and handle any medical issues, routine medical check-ups are essential. This could entail keeping an eye on cardiovascular health and electrolyte levels.

5. Support Teams:

• Participating in online or in-person support groups helps foster a feeling of belonging and understanding. Support groups may be led by organizations that specialize in eating disorders or by mental health experts.

6. In-patient Care or Comprehensive Programs:

• Hospitalization or enrollment in intense outpatient or inpatient treatment programs may be required in extreme circumstances. These programs offer more regimented and focused care, frequently combining medical supervision, counseling, and nutritional assistance.

7. Treatment Based on Family (FBT):

• FBT includes the family in the healing process, particularly when treating teenagers. It gives parents the confidence to actively aid in their child's rehabilitation.

8.   Interventions   with Mindfulness and Body Image:

• To encourage self-awareness, self-compassion, and a better relationship with one's body, treatments may include strategies like mindfulness and body image therapies.

9. Preventing Relapses:

• Create and put into action relapse prevention techniques, such as continued counseling, support groups, and a customized strategy for upholding a healthy lifestyle.

It's crucial to remember that the patient's dedication and active engagement are key components of therapy success. The keys to bulimia nervosa recovery are thorough treatment and early intervention. People should collaborate closely with a medical team to create a personalized treatment plan that takes into account their particular requirements and obstacles. It's critical to get professional assistance as soon as possible if you or someone you know is exhibiting bulimia symptoms.

CHAPTER THREE
Journey of Recovery

Every person's road to recovery from bulimia nervosa is different and may include a number of phases, difficulties, and victories. Here are a few crucial elements of the healing process:

1. Recognizing the Issue:

• An important first step in treating bulimia nervosa is recognizing and accepting its presence. This could entail getting over denial and realizing that the illness is having an impact on one's physical and mental health.

2. Getting Expert Assistance:

• It's crucial to speak with medical specialists, such as a primary care physician, therapist, psychiatrist, or nutritionist. Experts are qualified to do evaluations, offer diagnoses, and direct patients toward suitable courses of action.

3. Formulating a Course of Treatment:

• Working together to create a customized strategy with a treatment team is essential. This could involve medical supervision, dietary advice, psychotherapy, and, in certain situations, medication.

4. Counseling and Psycho therapy:

• Attending psychotherapy, especially evidence-based methods such as cognitive-behavioral therapy (CBT), can assist people in examining and altering maladaptive patterns of thinking and behavior about food, body image, and self-worth.

5. Rehabilitation of Nutrition:

• It is crucial to develop regular and balanced eating patterns in collaboration with a trained dietitian or nutritionist. A part of the process involves learning to enjoy a variety of foods in moderation.

6. Management of Medication:

• Following a doctor's orders and taking medication as given on a regular basis will help control symptoms and promote healing.

7. Putting Together a Support Network:

• Including loved ones and friends in the healing process can be a great source of support. Participating in live or virtual support groups enables people to establish connections with like-minded persons who can relate to their experiences.

8. Acquiring Coping Techniques:

• It's critical to develop healthier coping strategies to handle stress, emotions, and obstacles in life. This could entail picking up and using mindfulness practices, stress-reduction methods, and effective communication tactics.

9. Resolving Fundamental Problems:

• An essential part of treatment is identifying and treating any underlying emotional, psychological, or interpersonal problems that might be causing the eating disorder.

10. Creating Reasonable Objectives:

• Setting short- and long-term, realistic, and attainable goals is crucial for keeping motivation high and monitoring advancement.

11. Preventing Relapses:

• Creating a plan to prevent relapses is crucial to overcoming possible obstacles. This could entail pinpointing triggers, spotting early warning indicators, and putting plans in place to stop reverting to disordered behavior.

12. Honoring Successes:

• Marking and commemorating significant anniversaries and victories in the healing process can inspire and bolster constructive adjustments.

13. Persistent Self-Care:

• Sustained healing requires embracing a holistic approach to health, which takes into account one's mental, emotional, and physical well-being. Regular self-care practices improve general wellness. These practices include getting enough sleep, exercising, and having leisure time.

It is imperative to underscore that the process of recovery is dynamic and continuous. Relapses are possible, but they can also present chances to develop and improve coping mechanisms. Three essential components of the healing process from bulimia nervosa are tenacity, self-compassion, and patience. Seeking expert advice and assistance is essential for long-term improvement if you or someone you know is embarking on this journey.

Handling Challenges and Triggers

Managing obstacles and triggers is an essential part of the bulimia nervosa recovery process. A more successful and long-lasting rehabilitation may result from recognizing and controlling triggers as well as from creating efficient coping mechanisms. The following are some techniques for overcoming obstacles and triggers:

1. Determine Triggers:

• Consider particular circumstances, feelings, or occurrences that might set off bulimia-related ideas or actions.

Stress, social settings, body dissatisfaction, or unpleasant feelings are typical triggers.

2. Raise Your Minds:

• Develop self-awareness to spot early indicators of distress or the start of negative ideas and actions. Remaining in the present moment can be facilitated by practicing mindfulness.

3. Talk Honestly:

• Develop open lines of communication with the members of your treatment team, such as the dietitians, therapists, and medical professionals. Talking about obstacles and triggers enables them to offer specialized support and direction.

4. Establish a Support Network:

• Encircle yourself with peers, relatives, and friends who are understanding and have been through similar experiences. Tell them about your struggles and triggers so they can offer support and encouragement when you need it.

5. Create Coping Mechanisms:

• Create a toolkit of coping mechanisms in collaboration with your therapist. These could be journaling, art therapy, deep breathing exercises, mindfulness, or relaxing activities that make you happy.

6. Make a Plan to Prevent Relapses:

• Work with your treatment team to create an extensive plan for preventing relapses. To stop a relapse into disordered behaviors, this plan should address trigger management, early warning sign detection, and coping mechanism implementation.

7. Establish Sensible Objectives:

• Divide long-term recuperation objectives into more doable, smaller measures. Reaching modest objectives can increase drive and self-assurance, which makes taking on bigger problems easier.

8. Fight Back Against Negative Ideas:

• Focus on recognizing and combating negative thought patterns pertaining to one's own value and body image. When it comes to treating distorted thinking, cognitive-behavioral therapy (CBT) is very successful.

9. Exercise Self-Compassion:

• Treat yourself with kindness as you heal. Recognize that failures can happen, but take use of the chance to grow and modify your tactics.

10. Limit Your Contact with Triggers:

• Try to limit your exposure to circumstances or settings that cause negative ideas or actions. You may need to set up healthy boundaries for your own wellbeing.

11. Seek Expert Assistance:

• Seek quick assistance from your treatment team or a mental health professional if difficulties become too much to handle. An early intervention can stop a recurrence.

12. Continue Your Treatment:

• Regularly show up for dietary counseling, therapy sessions, and doctor's visits. Maintaining participation in treatment offers continuing assistance and direction.

13. Honor Advancement:

• Celebrate and acknowledge every accomplishment, no matter how tiny. Honoring accomplishments can increase confidence and reward positive behavior.

14. Develop Healthier Lifestyle Practices:

• Adopt a healthy, balanced lifestyle that includes frequent exercise, enough rest, and a balanced diet. These routines support resilience and general well-being.

Rehab is a journey with ups and downs, so keep that in mind. Help is OK to ask for, and development is frequently not linear. People can better manage their recovery and provide the groundwork for long-term wellbeing by proactively addressing their triggers and obstacles.

CHAPTER FOUR
Developing Consistent Eating Routines

Developing consistent eating habits is essential to bulimia nervosa rehabilitation. Regular eating that is well-balanced helps lower the risk of binge episodes, control blood sugar levels, and improve mental and physical health in general. The following techniques can help you create consistent eating habits:

1. Organizing Meals:

• Collaborate with a nutritionist or licensed dietitian to develop a customized, well-balanced meal plan. For optimal nutrition, schedule regular meals and snacks throughout the day.

2. Organizing Your Diet:

• Create a regular eating routine by having meals and snacks at approximately the same times every day. This lessens the chance of impulsive eating and helps control hunger.

3. Incorporate Every Food Group:

• Make sure to incorporate a range of dietary types into your meals, such as fruits, vegetables, proteins, fats, and carbs. A well-balanced diet promotes general health and vitality.

4. Consciously Consuming Food:

• Eat mindfully by being aware of your body's signals of hunger and fullness. When dining, stay away from screens and work so that you may enjoy the meal to the fullest.

5. Don't Miss Meals:

• Missing meals might make you feel more hungry and even encourage binge eating. If you want to keep your energy levels steady, try eating regular, well-balanced meals.

6. Arrange Snacks:

• Plan your snacks in between meals to avoid being overly hungry, which can lead to binge episodes. Select healthy snacks like whole-grain crackers, fruit, nuts, or yogurt.

7. Drinking plenty of water

• Drink water throughout the day to stay hydrated. Because dehydration and hunger can sometimes be mistaken for one another, it's critical to consume enough fluids.

8. Contest Food Regulations:

• Assist your treatment team in challenging and modifying any tight dietary guidelines or regulations. A healthier connection with food is facilitated by establishing flexibility in dietary choices.

9. Take Care of Food Fears:

• Expose yourself gradually to foods that could be difficult or cause anxiety. To guarantee a gentle and encouraging approach, this can be carried out with the assistance of a nutritionist or therapist.

10. Keep a Food Journal:

• Record meals, snacks, and eating-related emotions in a food journal. This might reveal trends and point out areas in need of development.

11. Support for Meals:

• If at all feasible, enlist the aid of loved ones, friends, or support groups while eating. Eating with a dinner partner can boost confidence and add enjoyment to the experience.

12. Preparing meals and cooking:

• Cooking and meal preparation activities can help you develop a good relationship with food. Try different flavors and dishes to add excitement to your meals.

13. Rehab-Related Affirmations:

• Make use of encouraging words or affirmations about getting well and creating a regular eating schedule. Remind yourself that maintaining your health and wellbeing depends on feeding your body.

14. Honor accomplishments:

• Honor each meal that goes well as a step toward your healing. No matter how tiny your accomplishments have been, acknowledge them and use positive reinforcement to boost your drive.

Recall that creating consistent eating habits takes time, and consulting with therapists, dietitians, and medical specialists is acceptable. Fostering a positive and long-lasting relationship with food is the aim, and patience and consistency are essential. If difficulties arise, talk about them with your treatment team so that tactics can be customized to meet your rehabilitation objectives.

Conclusion

In summary, treating the physical, psychological, and nutritional elements of bulimia nervosa is just one step in the complex process of recovering from the condition. Important aspects in the rehabilitation process include identifying the symptoms and indicators, getting expert assistance, and actively participating in evidence-based treatments.

- Nutritional counseling, psychotherapy, and occasionally medication are used as forms of treatment. Sustained recovery is aided by the building of regular eating patterns and the creation of coping mechanisms to deal with obstacles and triggers. In addition to a dedication to self-care, family and social support are essential components of the healing process.

• It's critical to approach recovery with self-compassion, patience, and an understanding that setbacks are possible. An important part of the recovery process is developing a healthy connection with food and one's body, acknowledging little achievements, and maintaining contact with a treatment team.

Seeking expert help is crucial if you or someone you love is experiencing bulimia nervosa. Specialists in eating disorders, mental health issues, and medical professionals can offer the support and direction required to begin the healing process.

Recall that healing is a personal, continuous process, and that every step you take in the right direction is a huge accomplishment. Bulimia nervosa can be overcome, and people can move toward a healthier, more rewarding life, with dedication, perseverance, and a network of supportive people.

THE END

Printed in Great Britain
by Amazon